YOGA *Journal*

GET FIT & STAY HEALTHY WITH YOGA

Speedy Publishing LLC
40 E. Main St., #1156
Newark, DE 19711

www.SpeedyPublishing.Co

Copyright 2014
978-1-63287-911-0
First Printed April 17, 2014

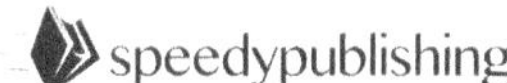

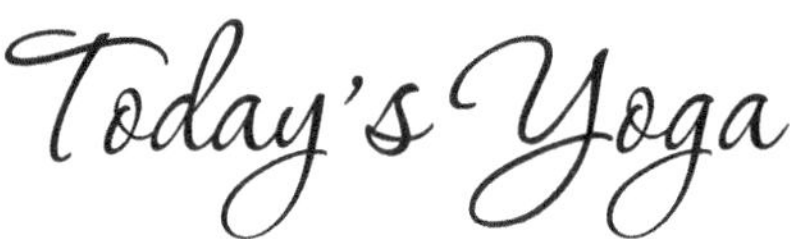

Today's Yoga

Date:

Before Yoga, I feel...

....

....

Today's Practice

Pose	Reps		Total Time

After Yoga, I feel...

....

....

Notes

....

....

....

....

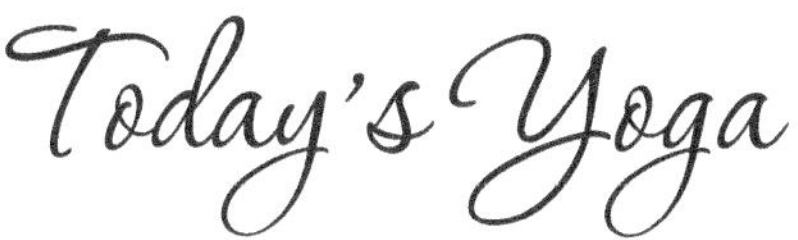

Today's Yoga

Date:

Before Yoga, I feel...

Today's Practice

Pose	Reps		Total Time

After Yoga, I feel...

Notes

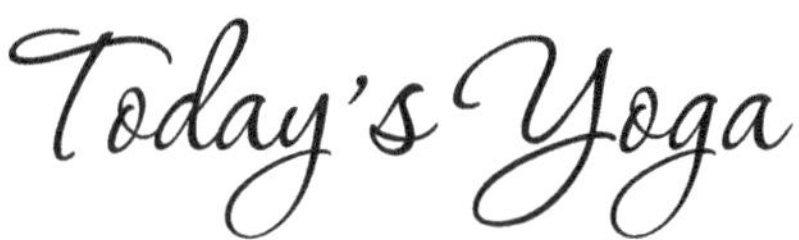

Today's Yoga

Date:

Before Yoga, I feel...

....

....

Today's Practice

Pose	Reps		Total Time

After Yoga, I feel...

....

....

Notes

....

....

....

Today's Yoga

Date:

Before Yoga, I feel...

....

....

Today's Practice

Pose	Reps		Total Time

After Yoga, I feel...

....

....

Notes

....

....

....

....

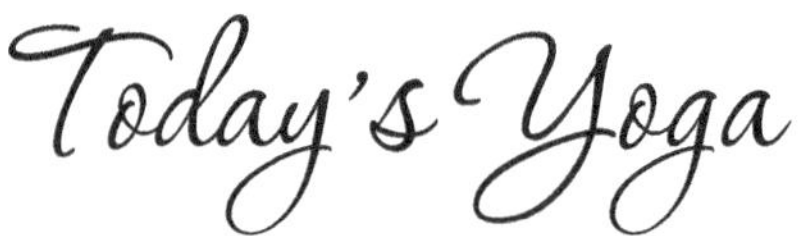

Today's Yoga

Date:

Before Yoga, I feel...

....

....

Today's Practice

Pose	Reps		Total Time

After Yoga, I feel...

....

....

Notes

....

....

....

....

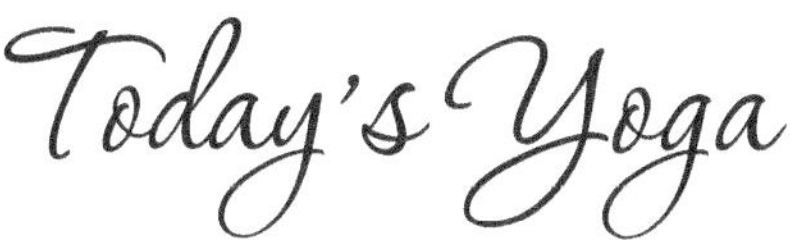

Today's Yoga

Date:

Before Yoga, I feel...

Today's Practice

Pose	Reps		Total Time

After Yoga, I feel...

Notes

Today's Yoga

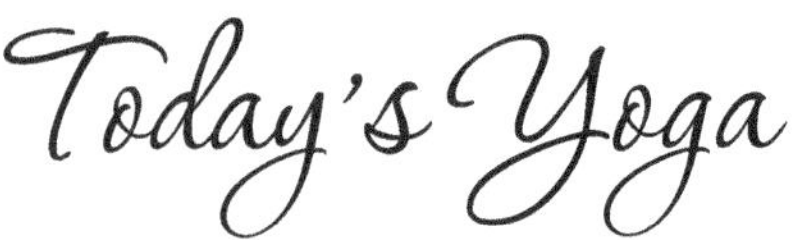

Date:

Before Yoga, I feel...

Today's Practice

Pose	Reps		Total Time

After Yoga, I feel...

Notes

Today's Yoga

Date:

Before Yoga, I feel…

....

....

Today's Practice

Pose	Reps		Total Time

After Yoga, I feel…

....

....

Notes

....

....

....

Today's Yoga

Date:

Before Yoga, I feel...

....

....

Today's Practice

Pose	Reps		Total Time

After Yoga, I feel...

....

....

Notes

....

....

....

Today's Yoga

Date:

Before Yoga, I feel...

....

....

Today's Practice

Pose	Reps		Total Time

After Yoga, I feel...

....

....

Notes

....

....

....

....

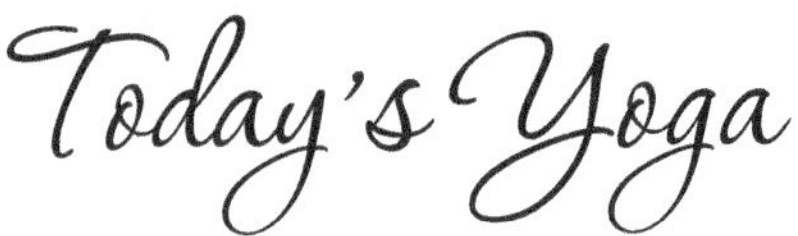

Today's Yoga

Before Yoga, I feel...

Today's Practice

Pose	Reps		Total Time

After Yoga, I feel...

Notes

Today's Yoga

Date:

Before Yoga, I feel...

Today's Practice

Pose	Reps		Total Time

After Yoga, I feel...

Notes

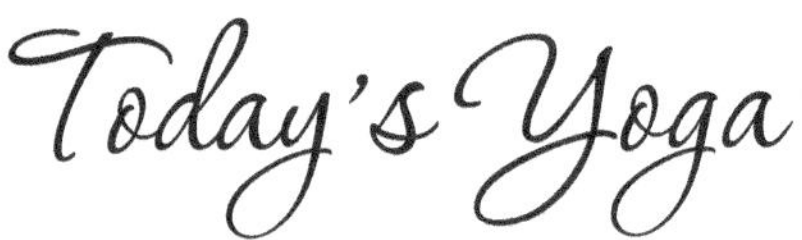

Today's Yoga

Date:

Before Yoga, I feel...

....

....

Today's Practice

Pose	Reps		Total Time

After Yoga, I feel...

....

....

Notes

....

....

....

....

Today's Yoga

Date:

Before Yoga, I feel...

....

....

Today's Practice

Pose	Reps		Total Time

After Yoga, I feel...

....

....

Notes

....

....

....

....

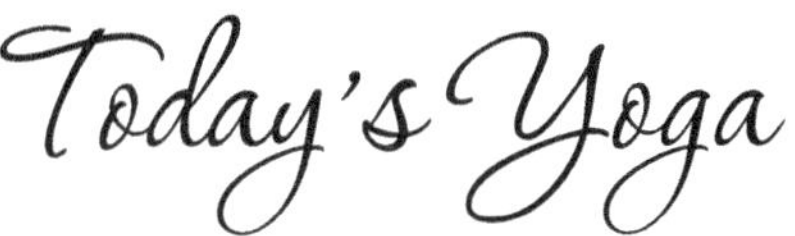

Today's Yoga

Date:

Before Yoga, I feel...

....
....

Today's Practice

Pose	Reps		Total Time

After Yoga, I feel...

....
....

Notes

....
....
....
....

Today's Yoga

Date:

Before Yoga, I feel...

....

....

Today's Practice

Pose	Reps		Total Time

After Yoga, I feel...

....

....

Notes

....

....

....

....

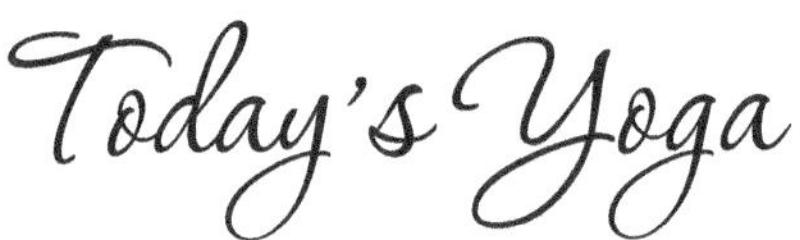

Today's Yoga

Date:

Before Yoga, I feel...

....
....

Today's Practice

Pose	Reps		Total Time

After Yoga, I feel...

....
....

Notes

....
....
....
....

Today's Yoga

Date:

Before Yoga, I feel...

Today's Practice

Pose	Reps		Total Time

After Yoga, I feel...

Notes

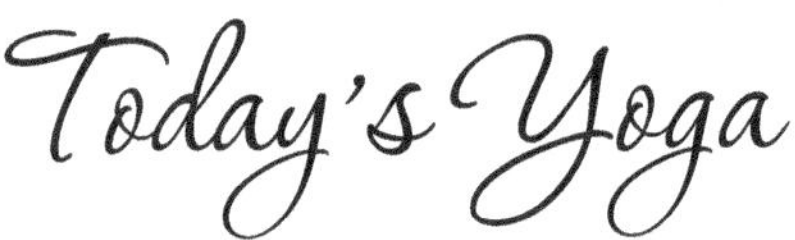

Today's Yoga

Date: [____]

Before Yoga, I feel...

....

....

Today's Practice

Pose	Reps		Total Time

After Yoga, I feel...

....

....

Notes

....

....

....

....

Today's Yoga

Date:

Before Yoga, I feel...

....

....

Today's Practice

Pose	Reps		Total Time

After Yoga, I feel...

....

....

Notes

....

....

....

....

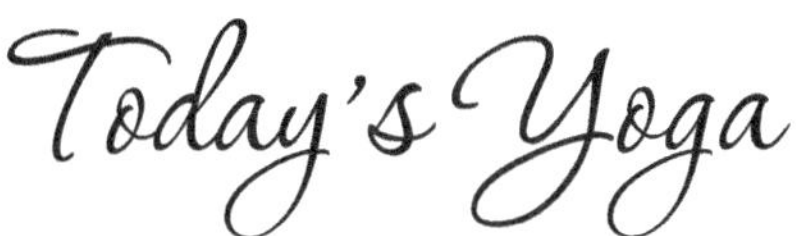

Today's Yoga

Date:

Before Yoga, I feel...

....

....

Today's Practice

Pose	Reps		Total Time

After Yoga, I feel...

....

....

Notes

....

....

....

....

Today's Yoga

Date:

Before Yoga, I feel...

Today's Practice

Pose	Reps		Total Time

After Yoga, I feel...

Notes

Today's Yoga

Date:

Before Yoga, I feel...

Today's Practice

Pose	Reps		Total Time

After Yoga, I feel...

Notes

Today's Yoga

Date:

Before Yoga, I feel...

Today's Practice

Pose	Reps		Total Time

After Yoga, I feel...

Notes

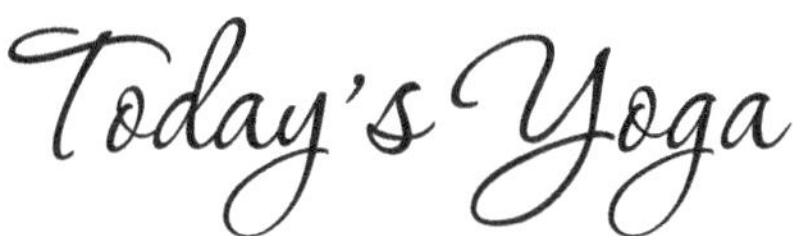

Before Yoga, I feel...

Today's Practice

Pose	Reps		Total Time

After Yoga, I feel...

Notes

Today's Yoga

Date:

Before Yoga, I feel...

Today's Practice

Pose	Reps		Total Time

After Yoga, I feel...

Notes

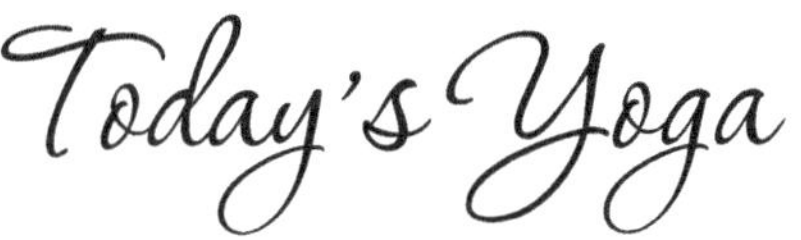

Today's Yoga

Date:

Before Yoga, I feel...

....
....

Today's Practice

Pose	Reps		Total Time

After Yoga, I feel...

....
....

Notes

....
....
....
....

Today's Yoga

Date:

Before Yoga, I feel...

Today's Practice

Pose	Reps		Total Time

After Yoga, I feel...

Notes

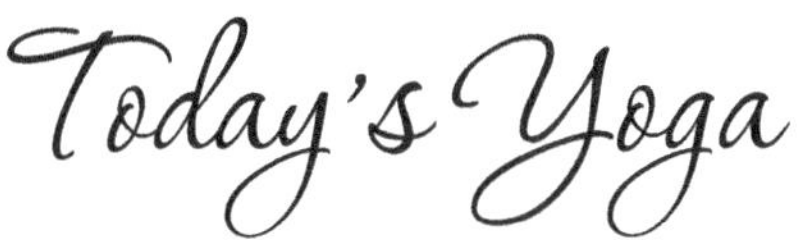

Today's Yoga

Date:

Before Yoga, I feel...

....

....

Today's Practice

Pose	Reps		Total Time

After Yoga, I feel...

....

....

Notes

....

....

....

....

Today's Yoga

Date:

Before Yoga, I feel...

....

....

Today's Practice

Pose	Reps		Total Time

After Yoga, I feel...

....

....

Notes

....

....

....

....

Today's Yoga

Date:

Before Yoga, I feel...

Today's Practice

Pose	Reps		Total Time

After Yoga, I feel...

Notes

Today's Yoga

Date:

Before Yoga, I feel…

....

....

Today's Practice

Pose	Reps		Total Time

After Yoga, I feel…

....

....

Notes

....

....

....

....

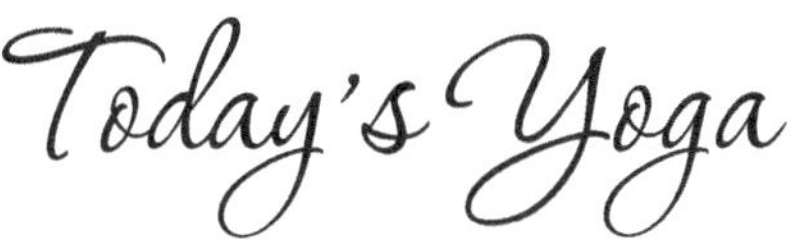

Today's Yoga

Date: ___________

Before Yoga, I feel...

....

....

Today's Practice

Pose	Reps		Total Time

After Yoga, I feel...

....

....

Notes

....

....

....

....

Today's Yoga

Date:

Before Yoga, I feel...

....

....

Today's Practice

Pose	Reps		Total Time

After Yoga, I feel...

....

....

Notes

....

....

....

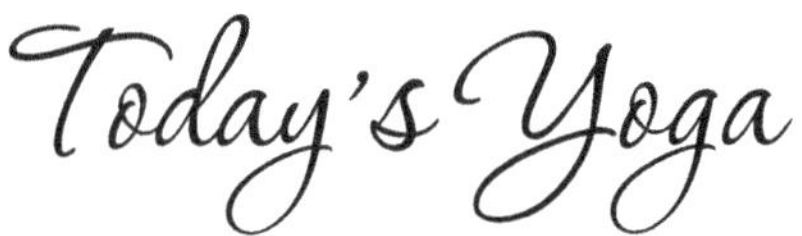

Today's Yoga

Date:

Before Yoga, I feel...

....

....

Today's Practice

Pose	Reps		Total Time

After Yoga, I feel...

....

....

Notes

....

....

....

....

Today's Yoga

Date:

Before Yoga, I feel...

....

....

Today's Practice

Pose	Reps		Total Time

After Yoga, I feel...

....

....

Notes

....

....

....

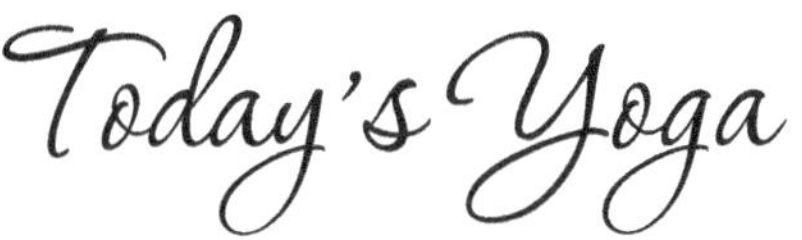

Today's Yoga

Date:

Before Yoga, I feel...

....

....

Today's Practice

Pose	Reps		Total Time

After Yoga, I feel...

....

....

Notes

....

....

....

....

Today's Yoga

Date:

Before Yoga, I feel...

....

....

Today's Practice

Pose	Reps		Total Time

After Yoga, I feel...

....

....

Notes

....

....

....

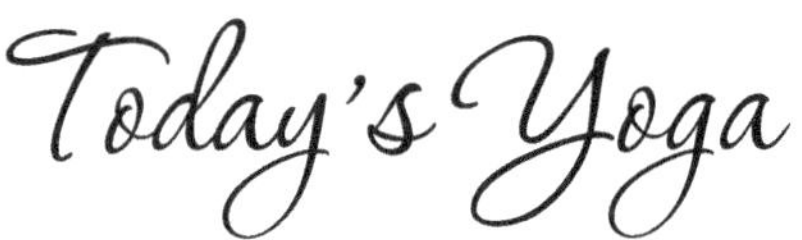

Today's Yoga

Date:

Before Yoga, I feel...

....

....

Today's Practice

Pose	Reps		Total Time

After Yoga, I feel...

....

....

Notes

....

....

....

....

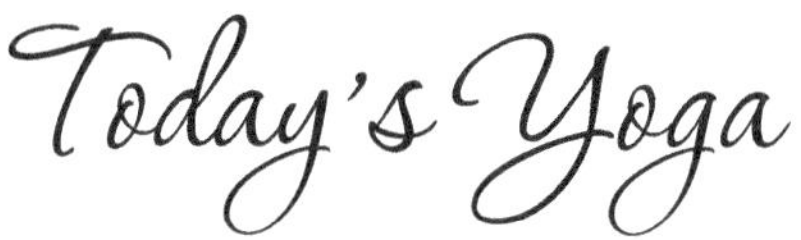

Today's Yoga

Date:

Before Yoga, I feel...

....
....

Today's Practice

Pose	Reps		Total Time

After Yoga, I feel...

....
....

Notes

....
....
....
....

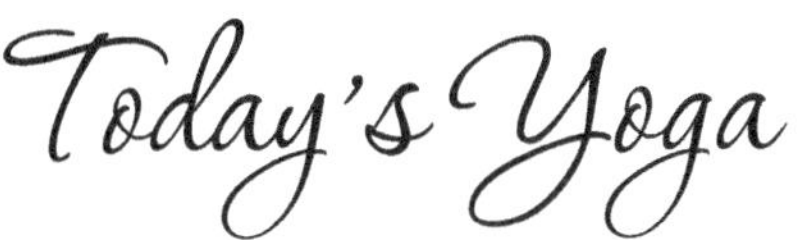

Today's Yoga

Date:

Before Yoga, I feel...

....
....

Today's Practice

Pose	Reps		Total Time

After Yoga, I feel...

....
....

Notes

....
....
....

Today's Yoga

Date:

Before Yoga, I feel...

....

....

Today's Practice

Pose	Reps		Total Time

After Yoga, I feel...

....

....

Notes

....

....

....

....

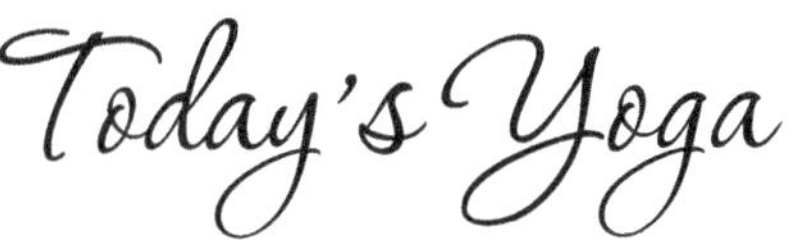

Today's Yoga

Before Yoga, I feel...

Today's Practice

Pose	Reps		Total Time

After Yoga, I feel...

Notes

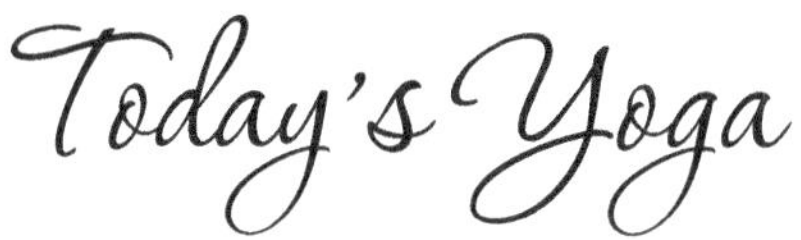

Today's Yoga

Date: ___________

Before Yoga, I feel...

....

....

Today's Practice

Pose	Reps		Total Time

After Yoga, I feel...

....

....

Notes

....

....

....

....

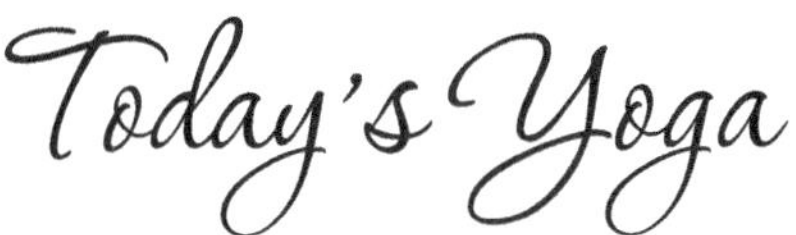

Today's Yoga

Date: ☐

Before Yoga, I feel...

....

....

Today's Practice

Pose	Reps		Total Time

After Yoga, I feel...

....

....

Notes

....

....

....

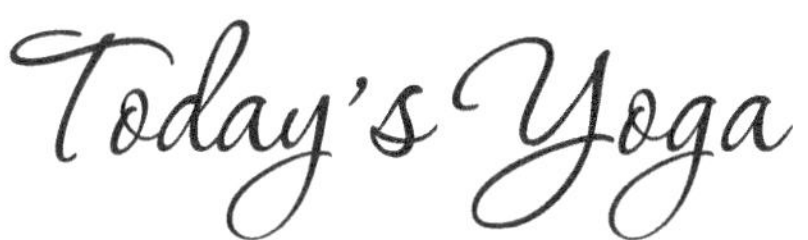

Today's Yoga

Before Yoga, I feel...

Today's Practice

Pose	Reps		Total Time

After Yoga, I feel...

Notes

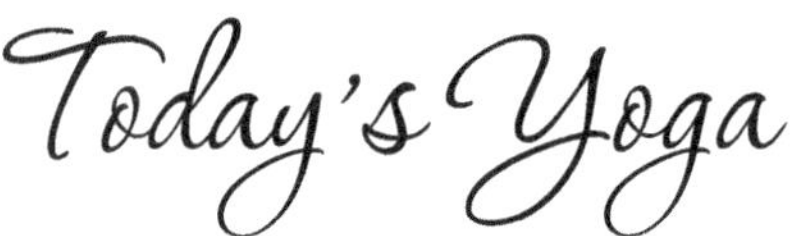

Today's Yoga

Date: ⬭

Before Yoga, I feel...

....

....

Today's Practice

Pose	Reps		Total Time

After Yoga, I feel...

....

....

Notes

....

....

....

....

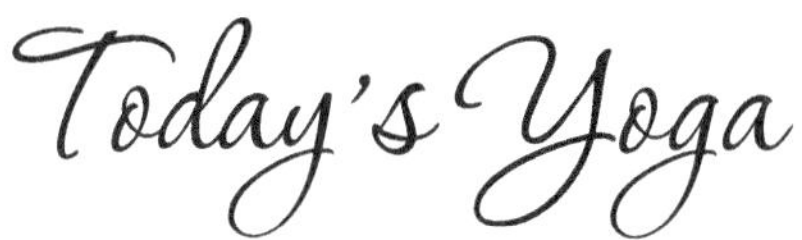

Today's Yoga

Date:

Before Yoga, I feel...

....

....

Today's Practice

Pose	Reps		Total Time

After Yoga, I feel...

....

....

Notes

....

....

....

....